# CBD OIL:

## UNDERSTANDING THE HEALING POWER & HEALTH BENEFITS OF MEDICINAL CANNABIS

**COLIN FELTON**

**Copyright © 2019 Publishing. All Rights Reserved.**

No part of this publication may be reproduced, distributed, or transmitted in any form or by any means, including photocopying, recording, or other electronic or mechanical methods, or by any information storage and retrieval system without the prior written permission of the publisher, except in the case of very brief quotations embodied in critical reviews and certain other noncommercial uses permitted by copyright law.

# TABLE OF CONTENTS

Introduction ............................................................................................................................................ 4

Chapter 1: What is CBD Oil? ................................................................................................................ 6

Chapter 2: Difference Between CBD & THC? ................................................................................... 13

Chapter 3: Forms of CBD Oil ............................................................................................................. 19

Chapter 4: Seven Benefits and Uses of CBD Oil ............................................................................... 22

Chapter 5: Where to buy CBD Oil ..................................................................................................... 29

Chapter 6: Choosing the Right CBD Oil For You ............................................................................. 34

Conclusion .......................................................................................................................................... 39

# INTRODUCTION

CBD Oil has been steadily gaining in popularity and for good reason! This safe and effective remedy has become a staple supplement for many. So, what is CBD Oil? To start, "CBD" is the acronym for Cannabidiol, a promising canabinoid found in the hemp plant and in medical/recreational cannabis. It is the agricultural hemp plant that is used to make CBD oil. While you've likely heard of THC, a psychoactive cannabinoid also found in both plants, agricultural hemp contains less than 0.3% THC, making it non-psychoactive.

CBD has a long history of being used to alleviate the symptoms of health problems. Queen Victoria used cannabis for menstrual cramps in the 19th century. Animal studies had long suggested that CBD lessens anxiety and reduces the severity and frequency of seizures, and today, this is a proven outcome on humans. The cannabis plant has been used for thousands of years in medicine for its sedative/hypnotic, antidepressant, analgesic, anticonvulsant, antiemetic, anti-inflammatory, anti-spasmodic, and appetite-stimulating effects.

The roots of CBD extend back thousands of years to the end of the first ice age. Archaeological finds suggest the source plant for the CBD compound, cannabis sativa, was likely one of the first agricultural crops planted by early man. In fact, growing cannabis sativa, something we tend to think of as modern, is often associated with the birth of agriculture 10,000 to 12,000 years ago.

The astronomer Carl Sagan, an icon of scientific credibility, put forth the possibility that Cannabis may have been the world's first agricultural crop, leading to the development of civilization. Looking at timelines, it is clear that cannabis plants have been integral to mankind since earliest times.

Cannabis plants are exceptionally versatile. Both the seeds and cannabis oil were used for food in China as early as 6,000 BC. Two thousand years later, in 4,000 BC, there is evidence of textiles made from hemp (cannabis) used in both China and Turkestan. The influence of the plant seems to have been global. In 850, the Vikings transported hemp rope and seeds to Iceland, and by the year 900, Arabs were learning techniques for making paper from hemp. By 1000, Italians were using ropes made of hemp on their sailing ships.

Today, consumers are primarily interested in the healthful properties of cannabis compounds, and there is a long thread of cannabis applications for health running through all eras of history. Stories about the healing properties of hemp (cannabis) mention Greek philosophers, Herodotus, Napoleon, and other legendary figures. The physician for Nero's army, for example, included cannabis in his inventory. In 1563, the health benefits of cannabis were discussed in a report by Portuguese physician Garcia da Orta. A few years later, China's Li Shih-Chen documented the antibiotic and anti-nausea effects of cannabis.

In contrast to today's modern restrictions of growing cannabis sativa, in 1533, England's King Henry VIII actually fined farmers if they did not raise hemp for industrial use. Less than one hundred years later, settlers in Jamestown, Virginia began growing hemp plants for it's unusually strong fibre. Once the plant demonstrated its usefulness, it became illegal NOT to grow hemp in Virginia, USA.

# Chapter 1:
# WHAT IS CBD OIL?

Cannabidiol, better known as CBD oil, has become an accepted natural alternative for a variety of health-related issues. It's use as a substitute for over-the-counter pharmaceutical drugs has been rapidly growing over the last few years. Unlike most supplements, it can be used for a broad range of issues, from lowering high blood pressure to providing relief for the side-effects associated with cancer treatments. However, one of the least understood benefits of CBD oil is its possible effectiveness in treating some symptoms associated with alcohol and drug addiction.

### What Is CBD Oil and How Does It Work?

Cannabidiol is a naturally occurring non-psychoactive element found in the cannabis sativa plant. It is also found in certain strains of hemp, the tough fibrous part of the cannabis herb. CBD oil is made by extracting resin from the stalks of hemp or cannabis flowers then diluting it with a carrier oil, such as coconut or olive oil. Most of the CBD oil used for medicinal purposes comes from hemp.

Scientific studies and anecdotal evidence reveal that CBD oil is helpful in reducing the symptoms of a wide variety of ailments. Although some of the health issues may differ, recent studies have shown that the body's endocannabinoid system is the common thread. Named after the cannabis plant, the endocannabinoid system consists of receptors and molecules that inhabit the brain, organs, glands, and cells within the human body.

The endocannabinoid system performs different jobs in various parts of the central nervous system, with the overarching goal of creating a stable equilibrium throughout the human body. The balance that the endocannabinoid system maintains among tissues, organs, and cells enables the body's systems to perform at peak performance. Since endocannabinoid receptors have such a big job, they are viewed by scientists as the key to health and fitness. These hard-working receptors are responsible for regulating the following bodily functions:

- Memory
- Motor coordination
- Pain Perception
- Temperature Control
- Mood
- Sleep
- Bone growth
- Eye Pressure
- Nerve and brain tissue
- Immune Function
- Appetite and hunger
- Metabolism

Cannabinoids have a profound effect on the endocannabinoid system by acting directly and indirectly on the body's receptors. If the endocannabinoid system is weak, cannabinoids can help the receptors function at an optimum level. CBD helps cells connect with the central nervous system and organs to create a perfect balance between the body and mind.

### How Does CBD Differ From Marijuana?

Marijuana is the dried leaves, flowers, stems, and seeds of cannabis sativa. Cannabis contains Tetrahydrocannabinol (THC) and CBD. THC is the component in cannabis that causes the feeling of euphoria by interacting with CB1 receptors in the brain. These receptors affect coordination, mood, thinking, and appetite. THC's interaction with these receptors induces the result typically connected with the use of marijuana that's associated with the sensation of "getting high." Unlike THC, cannabinoids are non-psychoactive, and their interaction with the CB1 receptors does not alter impressions, awareness, or judgment. Although CBD oil does not modify perception, it does create changes in the body that are essential to maintaining good health and wellness. Overall, CBD oil pulls out the useful compounds found in cannabis, without the psychoactive chemicals that produce the effects associated with inhaling marijuana.

### CBD Oil Benefits List

CBD oil has become quite popular for individuals looking for relief from pain and other ailments but don't feel comfortable using pharmaceutical drugs. Because of the way cannabinoids interact with the body, CBD oil has a variety of uses. Here are some common ailments that CBD oil has shown success in treating.

- Alleviating chronic pain
- Reducing cancer-related symptoms
- Improving heart health
- Treating acne and other skin conditions
- Reducing childhood epileptic seizures
- Treating inflammation

- Neutralizing free radicals

The CBD oil benefits list addresses a wide range of health issues that many people deal with daily. But research has shown that cannabinoids may be effective in treating symptoms associated with anxiety and depression.

**CBD Oil For Anxiety And Depression**

Anxiety and depression are recurrent mental health issues that have a debilitating impact on quality of life. Both ailments are typically treated with prescribed drugs that can have unpleasant side effects, such as sexual dysfunction and insomnia. In addition, some pharmaceutical drugs can be addictive and lead to substance abuse.

CBD helps to regulate the internal functions within the body and regulate the mind's external responses to the environment. Several studies have shown that CBD oil may be a feasible treatment for depression and anxiety. This has encouraged many people living with mental health issues to seek CBD oil as an alternative treatment. CBD binds to the body's serotonin receptors, causing a decrease in feelings of anxiety and depression.

There is no miracle cure for anxiety and depression. However, several case studies and clinical trials have shown that cannabinoids help regulate mood and emotions. This is why CBD oil is becoming a useful option for the ongoing management of some mental health disorders. More research is needed to gauge the efficacy of its uses for treating anxiety and depression. Anyone considering using CBD oil to treat mental health disorders should always consult with their doctor first.

### CBD Oil For Addiction Recovery

Compelling scientific evidence has revealed that CBD oil may be an effective method for treating some substance abuse related symptoms. As with most chronic illnesses, addiction is a disease that may have episodes of relapse and remission. The Substance Abuse and Mental Health Services Administration reported, in 2014, 21.5 million Americans were in need of therapeutic treatment for addiction. Because CBD is not addictive and is non-psychoactive, it may serve as the panacea for reducing cravings and anxiety experienced by individuals suffering from addiction. CBD's capacity to regulate the body's dopamine receptors is the key to providing relief for the following withdrawal symptoms:

- Excessive hunger
- Sleep issues
- Lethargy
- Muscle pain
- Disorientation and mental confusion
- Nausea
- Agitation and mood swings
- Cold and sweaty outbreaks

A recent study with animals by the Scripps Research Institute in San Diego discovered the brain's serotonin receptors are ignited by CBD. This was found to be directly related to a reduction in drug-seeking behavior. In this study, CBD oil was administered to rats after they were given alcohol and cocaine. The results indicated that, even five months after CBD had left their systems, the rats did not engage in drug-seeking behaviors.

CBD oil has also proven effective in breaking the smoking habit. The University of London conducted a study that found a relationship between cannabinoids and addiction to nicotine. In this study, habitual smokers were given an inhaler filled with CBD and a placebo. The participants who used the CBD inhaler showed a radical reduction in tobacco consumption, and their craving for nicotine decreased.

**Is CBD Oil Safe?**

Due to its association with marijuana, many ask the question, "Is CBD oil safe?" Although uncommon, some people have reported minor side-effects from using CBD oil. These include dry mouth, low blood pressure, feeling sleepy and light-headed. Although CBD is not toxic, always consult a healthcare professional before consuming the oil to treat chronic health conditions. This is essential for those who are pregnant, breastfeeding, or taking any prescribed medication.

**Administering CBD Oil**

Although many states have made the use of marijuana legal, most doctors are wary of prescribing CBD, due to the absence of an established guideline for recommended dosages. In fact, scientists have just recently started developing guidelines for administering medical marijuana. Therefore, determining the proper dosage of CBD oil depends on a variety of factors. Every individual is genetically unique, so a serving size of CBD oil will be different for each person. Again, it is recommended that you talk to a healthcare professional when considering dosage amounts for CBD.

CBD oil is usually taken orally in the form of drops or a paste. It is dispensed and held under the tongue until fully absorbed. It has a distinct flavor that some find unappealing, so drinking juice while ingesting the oil may be necessary. Other forms of oral administration include capsules, edible chocolate bars, and oral sprays. The diverse methods in which CBD oil can be consumed make it an appealing natural supplement that can be tailored to individuals' specific needs.

Due to the manner in which CBD oil interacts with the endocannabinoid system, there are many significant benefits from using it as a natural supplement. Recent studies have shown promising results in the efficacy of cannabinoids as a therapeutic treatment for many ailments. Scientific and anecdotal evidence has revealed that CBD oil is a safe and non-toxic alternative to some prescription drugs. This non-psychoactive supplement has proven to be a viable option for reducing the symptoms of an assortment of chronic ailments and diseases.

# Chapter 2:
# DIFFERENCE BETWEEN CBD AND THC?

As the debate of legalizing marijuana continues to rage on, the difference between key compounds in cannabis, CBD and THC, is becoming increasingly important. They both have very different effects and uses that range from recreational to medically groundbreaking.

You may have heard of cannabidiol oil (thanks to novelty products like CBD dog treats and vapes), but when talking about legal marijuana, it's important to note key distinctions. Despite varying public opinion on marijuana, these two separate compounds (CBD vs. THC) have specific uses, most notably in the medical sphere. The advocacy of many medical professionals has helped the compound CBD garner support for legalization and further research.

As the wave of legalization of marijuana slowly hits, products derived from compounds CBD and THC have huge marketing, investment, and medical potential. But what is the difference between the two?

**What Is The Difference Between CBD & THC?**

The main difference between CBD (cannabidiol) and THC (tetrahydrocannabinol) is that CBD does not induce a high, whereas THC does. Despite CBD and THC sharing a near exact molecular formula of $C_{21}H_{30}O_2$, and molecular mass of 314.469 g/mol and 314.464 g/mol, respectively, the compounds react quite differently.

THC, the psychoactive component of marijuana, induces sleep or drowsiness (a common effect of most strains of marijuana), whereas CBD keeps you awake and increases energy. And THC is responsible for the feeling of being high or body-high.

When reacting together, CBD actually works against the effects of THC by reducing anxiety, stress, or other negative feelings. For this reason, CBD is often extracted to use separately for non-psychoactive (and non-recreational) purposes.

**What Is CBD?**

CBD is only one of around 400 compounds in marijuana and is responsible for counteracting the effects of THC. Although the CBD molecule is almost identical to the THC molecule, it doesn't get you high. On its own, CBD has been proven to have many health benefits and uses, such as treating anxiety, stress, epilepsy, and depression. The compound is non-psychoactive, which has helped it gain support in many medical fields for its therapeutic properties.

It's benefits have been maximized by the retail and medicinal markets, with CBD products including oils, vapes, medicines, skincare, and drinks. Cannabinoid oil is a popular product created from CBD.

CBD has even been used for dogs to treat conditions like anxiety, mobility, pain, and heart disease. Products like dog treats and oils have become increasingly popular in recent years and are often recommended by veterinarians. CBD's antibiotic properties have also been linked to helping fight infections, although research results are mixed and inconclusive.

### Side Effects of CBD

Based on current research, side effects of CBD are rather limited. According to studies done by Medical Marijuana Inc., reports of drowsiness, dry mouth, and low blood pressure exist, but no links to serious side effects have been found.

### What is THC?

THC, or tetrahydrocannabinol, is a psychoactive component of marijuana, although the THC molecule is surprisingly similar to its non-psychoactive counterpart, CBD. THC gets you high and, for that reason, is somewhat less accepted for medicinal use than CBD.

Still, THC brags its own beneficial uses. THC has properties known to help treat pain, nausea, asthma, and even anorexia nervosa. However, as a psychoactive compound, its medicinal uses are still controversial.

### Side Effects of THC

In high-concentrations of THC, common negative side effects include reduced cognitive functions, anxiety, paranoia, dry mouth, red eyes, lethargy, and increased appetite. The positive effects of THC include increased relaxation, joint and headache relief, among others. It's worth noting that the increased appetite effect is often looked at as a benefit among chemotherapy patients suffering extreme loss of appetite, as well as individuals suffering from an eating disorder.

### Health Benefits of CBD vs. THC

The health benefits of CBD have been widely researched. With its non-psychoactive status, CBD has been known to treat health problems, most notably epilepsy. In a notice through the Federal Register in 2017, U.S. Food and Drug

Administration Deputy Commissioner Anna K. Abram claimed: "CBD has been shown to be beneficial in experimental models of several neurological disorders, including those of seizure and epilepsy."

It is clear that the positive benefits of compounds like CBD are becoming increasingly uncovered. The FDA is aware that "marijuana or marijuana-derived products are being used for a number of medical conditions including, for example, AIDS wasting, epilepsy, neuropathic pain, treatment of spasticity associated with multiple sclerosis, and cancer and chemotherapy-induced nausea," according to their website. Still, the use of many medical marijuana and CBD products are still awaiting official approval.

THC, while not used for as many applications as CBD, brags quite a few health benefits. In cannabis-oil form, studies have shown that THC can be used to treat neurodegenerative disorders, including Alzheimer's and Parkinson's. These studies also showed that THC can ease pain and help alleviate multiple sclerosis.

**CBD vs. THC For Anxiety**

Both THC and CBD have been used to treat anxiety. CBD has been used as an anxiolytic, or anxiety-treating drug, with some success. Studies show its potential to treat not only anxiety but also depression, PTSD, and obsessive-compulsive disorder.

However, THC has mixed reviews when treating anxiety. Due to its psychoactive nature, THC has been linked to feelings of anxiety or paranoia (perhaps most commonly experienced during marijuana use). However, the level or concentration of THC present is largely responsible if the consumer feels anxious, so the appropriate dose is the key.

## Negative Effects

While the jury is still out in some ways, studies so far have shown relatively few negative side effects of CBD and THC use. However, some studies show the neurotransmission systems involved in processing CBD can be linked to cannabis addiction and dependence and found links to the three stages of addiction. Positive effects were also found in the study.

Additionally, the THC compound in marijuana can have varying effects on stimulating anxiety. Studies have shown increased anxiety with marijuana use, but results vary depending on the individual's preconditions to anxiety or paranoia.

## Legality of CBD Vs. THC

The legality of both CBD and THC has been up for debate for quite a while. Apart from the nationwide debate (some may argue worldwide) on the legalization of marijuana, CBD's health benefits are still largely untapped due to FDA regulations.

In fact, the Drug Enforcement Administration (DEA) has attempted several times, more recently in 2016, to classify both THC and CBD as Schedule I drugs under the U.S. Controlled Substances Act, meaning they have "no currently accepted medical use and a high potential for abuse."

Despite such resistance, medical data and research continues to flood in in favor of legalizing components such as CBD for widespread use. However, CBD is illegal in all 50 states as of the writing of this article. Although the 2014 Farm Bill semi-legalized hemp production, it only covered a small set of hemp cultivation opportunities, such as for academic and researching purposes.

THC is often linked with marijuana in legality. As of 2018, medical marijuana is legal in 28 states plus Washington, D.C. However, the legality of purchasing or using THC is still a bit convoluted -- it only applies to states that have already made medicinal or recreational marijuana legal.

Although a bit of a blurred line, it is smart to be cautious when purchasing or using CBD products, as their legality is still questionable. The same goes for THC, which is perhaps the more controversial compound of the two for legal use.

### CBD Investment Opportunity

CBD has been used for products from oils to beverages, but most recently, it is a component of an epilepsy medication called Epidiolex, awaiting FDA approval. If approval is obtained, the over $1 billion marijuana industry could have huge investment potential. Several companies have begun buying out producers of cannabis in anticipation, notably Scott's Miracle-Gro Co.

The ruling on the FDA approval of Epidiolex and the use of CBD in such drugs is set for the end of June 2019. Not only are we seeing an increase in the legalization of marijuana, but the medicinal benefits of compounds found in marijuana, such as CBD, have huge market and investment potential.

### Increasing Legalization of Marijuana

Both recreational and medical marijuana have had a huge upswing in approval ratings in recent years, according to Gallup polls. With more states legalizing its use, THC and CBD have potential for medicinal and production applications. And, with the huge marijuana market ready to be tapped, we should see greater investment potential in CBD-related manufacturing.

**Before you keep reading**...if you have learned something new already, take a quick moment to leave an honest review at http://bit.ly/Understand_CBD

# Chapter 3:
# FORMS OF CBD OIL

### What Are The Different Forms Of CBD?

There are three main types of CBD available on store shelves: oils, isolates, and wax. To confuse the issue further, each can be offered in one or more types of products: oils, tinctures, creams and gels, capsules, sublingual sprays, transdermal patches, or vapors.

The concentration, dosage, and benefits of CBD can vary by product, depending on the type of CBD and the extraction and manufacturing processes used. You also need to consider that different ways of consuming CBD affect its bioavailability (the amount of active substance absorbed by the body).

When you ingest CBD, it will take a while to feel the effects, as it has to go through the digestive system and circulate through the liver. During this process, the amount of CBD available for your body will be reduced, but this is also a way to get lasting effects.

Products applied under your tongue or inhaled are absorbed directly through the mucous membranes into the blood stream and are available to the body immediately.

Products containing CBD oil are widely available on the market. You can find it in capsules, tinctures, or added to edibles. It can also be added to a number of non-edible products, such as balms and lotions. These work well if you're looking for something to use topically to soothe rashes or sore muscles.

### CBD Wax

Wax comes in different forms and may be referred to as CBD shatter, live resin, crumble, or budder. It's produced by treating the extract so that it becomes solidified and crystallized.

This form of CBD is highly concentrated, and typically, people will ingest it via dabbing. Dabbing CBD wax is pretty potent and can provide instant relief from pain and other problems. But you should use it with caution, since the substance in this form is quite concentrated.

### CBD Isolate

All-natural CBD isolate is about as pure and natural as it gets. This is, in part, due to the production process, which eliminates the chance of trace amounts of THC or contaminants.

CBD isolate contains the actual amount of CBD as is in the product (e.g., 10 mg of isolate equals 10mg of CBD), which allows for accurate dosing. CBD isolate is used in many of the same products as those manufactured from oils. Both are easily dissolved in carrier oils.

### CBD Crystals or Sheets

CBD isolate may also be made into crystals or sheets. You may prefer to buy your CBD as pure crystals in order to choose how you prefer to ingest it. You can use crystals to make your own capsules, edibles, and creams.

You can also add them to food and drinks or sprinkle them on a cigarette. Crystals can also be used for dabbing, a method of inhaling that is becoming very popular, as it gives you a quick "hit" of the substance. Dabbing requires a special setup, where the substance is dabbed onto a nail that heats it and releases the vapour.

### E-Liquids

CBD liquids for vaping (some with nicotine and some with THC) are available for purchase on the market.

### CBD Supplements: What's Really in the Capsule?

Now you know a little about the many forms of CBD, but how are you to know if a product is quality, or even legit, before you buy? First, you should know the supplement industry is currently much less regulated than the CBD space.

### What does this mean?

It means that anyone can make a CBD supplement without formal regulation or testing. Though the cannabis industry is booming and will continue to do so, until there is official regulation and control of substances like CBD, you should do your research to have a clear understanding of what you're purchasing before you do so. But as long as your ask the right questions, it shouldn't be too hard to find the best vendors with premium products.

### Don't hesitate to reach out to vendors with questions like:

- Is this a full-spectrum or pure CBD oil, an extract, isolate, or wax?
- What is the actual quantity of CBD in the product?
- What is this product best used for?
- How was this product produced?
- Can you give me the name of the company that produced this product?
- Do you have any paperwork to show this product is authentic?
- Do you offer exchanges or refunds if I feel the product is not of the quality that is advertised?

# Chapter 4:

# SEVEN BENEFITS AND USES OF CBD OIL (PLUS SIDE EFFECTS)

Cannabidiol is a popular natural remedy used for many common ailments. Better known as CBD, it is one of the 104 chemical compounds known as cannabinoids found in the cannabis or marijuana plant, Cannabis sativa.

Tetrahydrocannabinol (THC) is the main psychoactive cannabinoid found in cannabis and causes the sensation of getting "high" that's often associated with marijuana. However, unlike THC, CBD is not psychoactive.

This quality makes CBD an appealing option for those who are looking for relief from pain and other symptoms, without the mind-altering effects of marijuana or certain pharmaceutical drugs.

CBD oil is made by extracting CBD from the cannabis plant then diluting it with a carrier oil, like coconut or hemp seed oil. It's gaining momentum in the health and wellness world, with some scientific studies confirming it may help treat a variety of ailments, like chronic pain and anxiety.

**Here are seven health benefits of CBD oil backed by scientific evidence.**

### 1. Relieve Pain

Marijuana has been used to treat pain as far back as 2900 B.C. More recently, scientists have discovered that certain components of marijuana, including CBD, are responsible for its pain-relieving effects.

The human body contains a specialized system, called the endocannabinoid system (ECS), which is involved in regulating a variety of functions, including sleep, appetite, pain, and immune system response.

The body produces endocannabinoids, which are neurotransmitters that bind to cannabinoid receptors in your nervous system. Studies have shown that CBD may help reduce chronic pain by impacting endocannabinoid receptor activity, reducing inflammation, and interacting with neurotransmitters.

For example, one study in rats found that CBD injections reduced pain response to surgical incision, while another rat study found that oral CBD treatment significantly reduced sciatic nerve pain and inflammation.

Several human studies have found that a combination of CBD and THC is effective in treating pain related to multiple sclerosis and arthritis.

An oral spray, called Sativex, which is a combination of THC and CBD, is approved in several countries to treat pain related to multiple sclerosis.

In a study of 47 people with multiple sclerosis, those treated with Sativex for one month experienced significant improvement in pain, as well as walking and muscle spasms, compared to the placebo group.

Another study found that Sativex significantly improved pain during movement, pain at rest, and sleep quality in 58 people with rheumatoid arthritis.

## 2. Reduce Anxiety and Depression

Anxiety and depression are common mental health disorders that can have devastating impacts on health and well-being. According to the World Health Organization, depression is the single largest contributor to disability worldwide, while anxiety disorders are ranked sixth.

Anxiety and depression are usually treated with pharmaceutical drugs that can cause a number of side effects, including drowsiness, agitation, insomnia, sexual dysfunction, and headache.

What's more, medications like benzodiazepines can be addictive and may lead to substance abuse. CBD oil has shown promise as a treatment for both depression and anxiety, leading many who live with these disorders to become interested in this natural approach.

In one study, 24 people with social anxiety disorder received either 600 mg of CBD or a placebo before a public speaking test. The group that received the CBD had significantly less anxiety, cognitive impairment, and discomfort in their speech performance, compared to the placebo group.

CBD oil has even been used to treat insomnia and anxiety safely in children with post-traumatic stress disorder. CBD has also shown antidepressant-like effects in several animal studies. These qualities are linked to CBD's ability to act on the brain's receptors for serotonin, a neurotransmitter that regulates mood and social behavior.

### 3. Alleviate Cancer-Related Symptoms

CBD may help reduce symptoms related to cancer and side effects related to cancer treatment, like nausea, vomiting, and pain.

One study looked at the effects of CBD and THC in 177 people with cancer-related pain, who did not experience relief from pain medication.

Those treated with an extract containing both compounds experienced a significant reduction in pain compared to those who received only THC extract. CBD may also help reduce chemotherapy-induced nausea and vomiting, which are among the most common chemotherapy-related side effects for those with cancer.

Though there are drugs that help with these distressing symptoms, they are sometimes ineffective, leading some people to seek alternatives.

A study of 16 people undergoing chemotherapy found that a one-to-one combination of CBD and THC administered via mouth spray reduced chemotherapy-related nausea and vomiting better than standard treatment alone.

Some test-tube and animal studies have even shown that CBD may have anticancer properties. For example, one test-tube study found that concentrated CBD induced cell death in human breast cancer cells. Another study showed that CBD inhibited the spread of aggressive breast cancer cells in mice. However, these are test-tube and animal studies, so they can only suggest what might work in people. More studies in humans are needed before conclusions can be made.

**4. Reduce Acne**

Acne is a common skin condition that affects more than 9% of the population. It is thought to be caused by a number of factors, including genetics, bacteria, underlying inflammation, and the overproduction of sebum, an oily secretion made by sebaceous glands in the skin.

Based on recent scientific studies, CBD oil may help treat acne due to its anti-inflammatory properties and ability to reduce sebum production. One test-tube study found that CBD oil prevented sebaceous gland cells from secreting excessive sebum, exerted anti-inflammatory actions, and prevented the activation of "pro-acne" agents, like inflammatory cytokines.

Another study had similar findings, concluding that CBD may be an efficient and safe way to treat acne due, in part, to its remarkable anti-inflammatory qualities. Though these results are promising, human studies exploring the effects of CBD on acne are needed.

## 5. Neuroprotective Properties

Researchers believe CBD's ability to act on the endocannabinoid system and other brain signaling systems may provide benefits for those with neurological disorders.

In fact, one of the most studied uses for CBD is in treating neurological disorders, like epilepsy and multiple sclerosis. Though research in this area is still relatively new, several studies have shown promising results. Sativex, an oral spray consisting of CBD and THC, has been proven to be a safe and effective way to reduce muscle spasticity in people with multiple sclerosis. One study found that Sativex reduced spasms in 75% of 276 people with multiple sclerosis, who were experiencing muscle spasticity that was resistant to medications.

In another study, researchers gave 214 people with severe epilepsy 0.9–2.3 grams of CBD oil per pound (2–5 g/kg) of body weight. Their seizures reduced by a median of 36.5%. One study found that CBD oil significantly reduced seizure activity in children with Dravet syndrome, a complex childhood epilepsy disorder, compared to a placebo.

However, it's important to note that some people in these studies experienced adverse reactions associated with CBD treatment, such as convulsions, fever, and diarrhea. CBD has also been researched for its potential effectiveness in treating several other neurological diseases.

For example, several studies have shown that treatment with CBD improved quality of life and sleep for people with Parkinson's disease. Additionally, animal and test-tube studies have shown that CBD may decrease inflammation and help prevent the neurodegeneration associated with Alzheimer's disease.

In one long-term study, researchers gave CBD to mice genetically predisposed to Alzheimer's disease, finding that it helped prevent cognitive decline.

### 6. Improve Heart Health

Recent research has linked CBD with several benefits for the heart and circulatory system, including the ability to lower high blood pressure.

High blood pressure is linked to higher risks of a number of health conditions, including stroke, heart attack, and metabolic syndrome. Studies indicate that CBD may be a natural and effective treatment for high blood pressure.

One recent study treated 10 healthy men with one dose of 600 mg of CBD oil and found it reduced resting blood pressure, compared to a placebo. The same study also gave the men stress tests that normally increase blood pressure. Interestingly, the single dose of CBD led the men to experience a smaller blood pressure increase than normal in response to these tests.

Researchers have suggested the stress- and anxiety-reducing properties of CBD are responsible for its ability to help lower blood pressure.

Additionally, several animal studies have demonstrated that CBD may help reduce the inflammation and cell death associated with heart disease due to its powerful antioxidant and stress-reducing properties. For example, one study found that treatment with CBD reduced oxidative stress and prevented heart damage in diabetic mice with heart disease.

### 7. Other Benefits

CBD has been studied for its role in treating a number of health issues other than those outlined above. Though more studies are needed, CBD is thought to provide the following health benefits:

- Antipsychotic effects: Studies suggest CBD may help people with schizophrenia and other mental disorders by reducing psychotic symptoms.
- Substance abuse treatment: CBD has been shown to modify circuits in the brain related to drug addiction. In rats, CBD has been shown to reduce morphine dependence and heroin-seeking behavior.
- Anti-tumor effects: In test-tube and animal studies, CBD has demonstrated anti-tumor effects. In animals, it has been shown to prevent the spread of breast, prostate, brain, colon, and lung cancer.
- Diabetes prevention: In diabetic mice, treatment with CBD reduced the incidence of diabetes by 56% and significantly reduced inflammation.

**Are There Any Side Effects?**

Though CBD is generally well-tolerated and considered safe, it may cause adverse reactions in some people. Side effects noted in studies include:

- Diarrhea
- Changes in appetite
- Fatigue

CBD is also known to interact with several medications. Before you start using CBD oil, discuss it with your doctor to ensure your safety and avoid potentially harmful interactions.

Can you or any of your loved ones use any of these seven benefits of CBD Oil to improve their health? Leave a review and share: http://bit.ly/Understand_CBD

# Chapter 5:
# WHERE TO BUY CBD OIL

Are you looking to buy CBD-rich oil? Finding the right CBD oil can be a daunting task, especially if you are a newbie. There are many ways to acquire your Cannabinoid (CBD) oil. You can purchase the product online, from brick and mortar stores, co-ops, dispensaries, and natural herbalists. CBD oil products can be made from extracts of either hemp plants or Marijuana Plants. Depending on your preferred mode of ingestion, the hemp-extracted oil is available in a range of applications, including tinctures, topicals, vaporizers, vape pens, transdermal patches, and as infused edibles.

### Raw

Raw CBD oil is exactly what it sounds like. Once the oil has been extracted, the oil does not go through any more processing and does not get filtered. Raw CBD oil can be green or dark in color because it often contains phytochemicals, chlorophyll, and raw plant material. Raw oil may contain impurities left over from the extraction process.

### Decarboxylated

Decarboxylated CBD oil means the CBD will be more active in the body. Decarboxylation is when the oil is heated to change the chemical components and "turn on" the CBD. This process improves the efficacy and potency of the oil, making it easier for the oil to have an impact on the body. Decarboxylated oil is often brown or darker in color.

### Filtered

Filtered oil has been through the most processing. Generally, filtered oil has been decarboxylated and then even further refined by filtering out the phytochemicals and plant materials. This makes the oil gold in color and is often considered the highest quality compared to raw or decarboxylated oil. Filtered oil is commonly referred to as "gold" CBD oil and is very popular among consumers. It also tends to be the most expensive, but this isn't always the case.

One of the important questions people will ask regarding CBD oil is whether it is legal to purchase. A vast majority of CBD oil is extracted from hemp, a non-psychoactive compound that contains none or a very low concentration of THC; hence, it is considered completely legal and separate from cannabis marijuana regulation and authority. Many states and countries around the world are changing their laws to legalize the use of medical marijuana. CBD hemp oil products can be shipped to 40 countries (including all 50 states of America) while those from marijuana plants are not legal in many states, nor can they be shipped across most state lines.

### Online Stores

Most CBD products are sold online. Buying online is a quick, convenient, and secure way to have your hemp oils and other CBD –based products delivered straight to your door. Whenever you buy products online, chances are the vendor will not offer just one particular product but a variety to choose from. You can choose from different variations and have the advantage of comparing prices of various merchants. Basically, you will quickly understand the landscape of the consumer market at the tap of a finger. The other great thing about buying online is that you can do research by going through reviews or social media to see what that particular provider's reputation is. If a particular vendor has many different complaints from different people, that should definitely raise a red flag. If you want to purchase the product online, it is advisable to study the potential benefits of the oils before you make the order. Beware of certain products that claim to be the perfect cure for everything. Any online store that promises to give you miracle oil that cures each and every problem is most likely a rip-off.

## Dispensaries

There is a growing number of medical cannabis dispensaries, offering CBD-rich products, in the U.S. Most physical dispensaries are required to operate under state health and safety standards set by law. The state conducts background checks on the owner and staff, and dispensaries must meet security requirements and strict licensing guidelines. When buying hemp-based CBD oil (low in THC or/and CBD), you will not need a card; however, to purchase cannabis plant-based CBD oil, patients need to be certified by a doctor who is part of their continuing care and who is registered with the state's medical-marijuana program. That, however, applies only to those living in states that have passed medical marijuana laws. It is important for one to visit the dispensaries and get information as to whether their products have been tested and undergone clinical trials.

## Brick and Mortar Stores

You can purchase CBD and hemp oil in specialty retail stores – over the counter (i.e., nutrition stores and smoke shops). Physical stores offer buyers the ability to see the products before they purchase, as well as the chance to engage with store associates by asking questions and learning about other products they might be interested in. When you are looking to choose a reputable and high-quality CBD retailer, it is also important to inquire about the product's third-party test results. This way, you will be assured that you are getting a high-quality and safe product, as reputable companies will invest in such tests to gain the trust of their customers.

Manufacturers are free to sell what they consider to be the best form of hemp oil CBD extract. This being the case, there are many companies taking advantage of the CBD oil demand, making products that don't contain enough or any CBD at all. All they care about is making profits by sourcing the cheapest CBD oils they can find on the market.

It's important to research in order to purchase the right product. Always use personal discretion when making purchases, both in-person and online. Further, don't always go for the cheap products but be willing to pay the price for a quality product. If you want to reap the benefits of excellent quality, you have no choice but to pay a substantial amount for it. Also, remember to check labels for any indication of the ingredients that make up the product, making sure it is hemp oil CBD. Any product that comes without a label or indication of ingredients is illegal and potentially dangerous. Even though no regulation exists, it is always good to take measures to ensure your own safety.

### Make the Right Choice

With no regulations when it comes to the distribution of CBD hemp-based products, you can never be sure what you are purchasing. This leaves consumers exposed to the side effects of impure hemp oil CBD. Despite these challenges, it is possible to buy the right CBD oil in the market. Several reputable companies have risen to offer reliable, safe, and potent CBD products to the market. Read reviews of the top selling CBD oils on our site to get an understanding of what makes them unique in this rapidly growing market, so you can make an informed decision. Our goal is to bring CBD to the people, while helping them make better decisions every day. You can count on us to provide CBD reviews you can trust. Keep in mind that we recommend only the best CBD brands on the market.

# Chapter 6:

# CHOOSING THE RIGHT CBD OIL FOR YOU

The medicinal cannabis industry is growing extremely fast. Although the large number of CBD oils available today is not a bad thing, it can make choosing the right product for you more difficult. Here is what you should consider before purchasing CBD oil.

With scientific research on the therapeutic potential of cannabis mounting and cannabis laws in many countries becoming more relaxed, it's not surprising the medicinal cannabis industry is exploding. Experts estimate the market for CBD oils and similar cannabidiol products to reach $13B USD. Sure, more products to choose from are a good thing for the consumer, but it doesn't necessarily make choices easier.

If you are a medicinal cannabis user or just looking to boost your overall health, the fact that you now have many different CBD oil products to choose from has its pros and cons.

On one hand, you can now legally obtain CBD oils in many regions, online or in retail stores. On the other hand, it can be challenging to find a CBD oil that is right for you. CBD oils are available in different concentrations and differ widely in the way they are made. Most importantly, the quality and purity of CBD oils, and therefore their effectiveness, vary from one manufacturer to another. Here are some tips on what you should look for when purchasing CBD oil.

### Choose a suitable concentration of CBD

CBD oil products, such as those offered in dropper bottles or capsule form, come in a range of concentrations. The amount of CBD they contain per bottle or capsule can usually be found on the packaging. Some list the amounts in mg, such as 250mg, 500mg, or 1,000mg. Other CBD oil products may specify the concentration as percentages, such as 4%, 10%, or 20% cannabidiol (CBD).

While higher doses of CBD will likely have a more pronounced effect, it is not recommended to start with a high concentration. Start with products featuring a low to moderate dosage then gradually work your way up to a higher dosage if needed. By observing the effects over the course of several days or a few weeks, you can make the necessary adjustments. If you don't see the desired effect after this period, increase your dosage. Once the desired effect sets in, you will be able to establish what concentration of CBD is best for you.

### Cost per dose can be a factor

Cost per dose is another factor to consider before purchasing CBD oil. Although highly concentrated products might be more expensive outright, they often offer a greater value over the life of the product. So, once you have established your therapeutic dose of CBD, see whether switching to a higher concentration saves you money in the long-run. For instance, a 500mg bottle of CBD oil will likely cost you less than if you were to buy two 250mg bottles.

### Full-spectrum CBD oil vs CBD isolate

The two main types of CBD oils are those made from near-pure CBD isolates or crystals and full-spectrum oils. The latter contains other active compounds in addition to CBD.

Until recently, pure CBD isolate was considered the standard for non-psychoactive cannabis therapy. But evidence is mounting that full-spectrum oils provide a host of additional benefits not seen in isolates. Full-spectrum oils often contain other cannabinoids, such as CBN and CBL, as well as terpenes (aromatic compounds such as pinene and limonene), and other substances like flavonoids. These compounds are said to work in synergy with CBD through a natural process known as the "entourage effect".

So, which one do you need?

Whether you should opt for a CBD oil made from CBD isolate or a full-spectrum oil is up to you. Both types offer benefits, but full-spectrum oils are currently the industry darling. When you purchase a CBD oil product, manufacturers usually state if their products are "full-spectrum" on the product page.

### Capsules or sublingual?

Almost as important as choosing the right concentration of CBD oil is the delivery method. Many CBD oils are available in dropper bottle form, allowing for sublingual delivery. This means dropping CBD oil directly under the tongue, making for an efficient route of delivery. Then again, capsules allow for discreet, controlled doses of CBD to be administered with ease.

Some individuals also inhale their CBD oils using vaporizers. These products may contain the same ingredients, but will differ when it comes to accessibility, convenience, and even effect. Conduct research on the different methods of intake to determine which route works best for you.

## Various extraction methods

There are various ways CBD is extracted from the cannabis plant to create CBD oils, and not all methods are created equal when it comes to the purity and quality of the final product. Some companies that cut corners and produce cheap CBD products may use harmful solvents, such as propane or butane, to render their extracts. Although these products are often less expensive, ask yourself if you really want to nullify the health benefits of the oil with products that contain remnants of harmful substances.

The best CBD oils are usually created via supercritical $CO_2$ extraction. This method uses carbon dioxide under high pressure to isolate, preserve, and maintain the purity of the CBD. It is admittedly more expensive to run, so the resulting products may not be the cheapest, but you can rest assured that you're buying a quality product. $CO_2$ extraction doesn't involve any toxic substances.

There are other, less common methods to extract CBD without the need for toxic substances. Olive oil or coconut oil can also be used to extract CBD, albeit less efficiently than $CO_2$.

Reputable manufacturers of CBD oils normally are quite transparent about their extraction processes. If you don't see extraction methods mentioned on the product page or any supplemental literature or packaging, proceed with caution. Those manufacturers that employ $CO_2$ extraction are often proud to mention it.

## Where does the CBD come from?

CBD oil is derived from hemp or cannabis plants—both of which belong to the same species of Cannabis sativa but have been selectively bred over the years to feature unique characteristics. Shadier CBD oil manufacturers are known to use non-food-grade hemp grown under non-organic and questionable conditions. This is bad since hemp is a plant that absorbs contaminants, such as chemicals, metals, lead etc, which will ultimately end up in your CBD oil.

Your best bet is to select from trusted European CBD oil manufacturers that source their cannabinoids, terpenes etc. from organic, non-psychoactive EU hemp. European regulations regarding hemp are very strict and ensure the highest-quality harvest. Combined with proper extraction and filtration methods, good raw material will result in oils of the utmost quality.

Once again, reputable manufacturers are usually quick to mention where their CBD is sourced from. Moreover, the best CBD oils are tested by professional third parties to ensure products are safe, high-quality, and contain what they claim.

These tests guarantee the product is free from pesticides, heavy metals, and other contaminants. If you can find the lab results on a product website, this is a good indication that the manufacturer takes quality and customer service seriously.

Before purchasing a CBD oil product, it is advised to scope out different companies and their offerings. Don't just look at the price of your CBD oil, and DO NOT buy from untrustworthy sources.

Stick to reputable European CBD oil manufacturers and you will be on the right track to incorporating the benefits of CBD into your lifestyle.

# CONCLUSION

Touted for a variety of health benefits, CBD is flooding the marketplace in the form of topicals, edibles, tinctures, and vape oils. If you're considering purchasing CBD oil, it's important to consider your health goals to determine the best form of CBD oil for you. For those seeking to promote restful sleep or relieve insomnia, consuming cannabidiol edibles or mixing tinctures into food or beverages is recommended.

Currently, there are no documented studies that show undesirable effects of CBD, which is why this particular cannabinoid is legal in most parts of the world. However, there are many studies showing CBD to cause only desirable effects or no effects at all. In virtually every test on CBD's effectiveness, only desirable effects were obtained; the only proven negative side effect is slight fatigue (and only when a lot of CBD was used). In fact, CBD has been extensively hailed by none other than Dr Sanjay Gupta, who discussed it at length in his documentary "Weed" on CNN live, as well as in a string of videos widely circulated on YouTube. CBD is now used to treat health conditions like neurological degeneration, for which no other successful medication has yet been found. CBD is suggested as a potentially useful therapy for schizophrenia due to its opposing effects. Not only that, but it may be able to relax those suffering from anxiety disorders and offer comfort.

If this book provided you with any new information or value regarding uses and benefits of CBD Oil, leave a review and share what you learned!
http://bit.ly/Understand_CBD

Made in the USA
Middletown, DE
01 March 2019